# *LOW IMPACT EXERCISE FOR MEN*

*6 minutes a Day Simple Workouts to Gain Flexibility Lose Weight, Improve Balance, Core strength and Independence With Ease*

Robert T. Wormley

# TABLE OF CONTENT

# INTRODUCTION

In a bustling metropolitan where the pace of life never stops, there lives a bright guy named Alex, whose zest for life knows no boundaries.

However, despite the excitement, Alex became trapped in the clutches of physical discomfort and health difficulties, a direct result of his sedentary employment and lifestyle.

The once-agile guy began to suffer from a lack of flexibility, knee stiffness, and constant back discomfort, all of which were caused by lengthy hours chained to his desk.

Alex realized the critical necessity for a revolutionary intervention as oncoming dangers loomed on the horizon. His concerns went beyond physical discomfort;

he was concerned about the subtle invasion of cardiovascular diseases, the burden of extra body weight, and the looming threat of chronic exhaustion and physiological weakness.

Driven by an unyielding determination to recapture his energy and resist his health's foreboding trend, Alex started on a search for knowledge and empowerment. In his search, he came upon a beacon of hope:

"Low Impact Exercise for Men," a book filled with specialized ideas and precisely detailed routines meant to energize the male physique while avoiding the drawbacks of high-impact activity.

With the zeal of a seeker on the verge of revelation, Alex dived into the book's wisdom, gathering pearls of advice and concrete ideas. Armed with fresh information, he set out on a road of change, smoothly incorporating the recommended workouts into the fabric of his everyday routine.

Days turned into weeks, and Alex witnessed a stunning mutation within his own being. The shackles of stiffness and soreness began to release, allowing for a renewed suppleness and vigor.

As each low-impact workout session progressed, Alex felt energy rushing through his veins, filling every muscle with fresh vigour and strength.

His devotion paid off in practical ways, as Alex experienced a revival of energy and vigor that pervaded every aspect of his life. No longer constrained by physical discomfort, he embraced life with renewed vigour and excitement, rejoicing in the freedom of movement and the thrill of unrestricted mobility.

Today, Alex exemplifies the transformational power of proactive health management as well as the unbreakable spirit of perseverance.

He has not only defeated the specter of discomfort and debilitation by incorporating low-impact exercise into his lifestyle, but he has also emerged as a beacon of encouragement for those looking to follow in his footsteps to holistic well-being.

 Alex's vivid tapestry exemplifies the triumph of mind over matter, as well as the limitless capacity of the human spirit to overcome hardship and embrace vitality with open arms.

# *Chapter 1: origin of Low Impact Exercise*

While low-impact exercise is a staple of current fitness routines, it has a centuries-long history. Its beginnings may be traced back to the understanding of the necessity of movement for health and well-being, particularly among men who want to maintain their physical fitness without putting their bodies under undue pressure or danger of injury.

Low-impact activities for males may be traced back to ancient civilizations like Greece and China, where Tai Chi and calisthenics were popular. These exercises stressed controlled movements, balance, and flexibility, laying the groundwork for low-impact fitness techniques that continue to this day.

The current notion of low-impact exercise gained popularity in the mid-twentieth century, owing to a growing knowledge of the advantages of cardiovascular health and the need for accessible fitness alternatives for all people, regardless of age or physical condition.

In the 1960s and 1970s, pioneers such as Jack LaLanne popularized low-impact workouts through television shows that emphasized swimming, strolling, and gentle stretching.

As the fitness industry evolved, so did the variety of low-impact workouts accessible for men. Aerobic exercises like cycling, elliptical training, and rowing have emerged as excellent techniques to enhance cardiovascular fitness while putting minimal strain on the joints.

Similarly, strength training routines using resistance bands, bodyweight movements, and light dumbbells became commonplace in low-impact workouts, allowing men to gain muscle and improve overall body composition safely and efficiently.

In recent decades, advances in exercise science and technology have increased the number of low-impact activities available to men. Suspension training systems, balancing boards, and low-impact cardio devices have opened up new possibilities for people to engage in difficult yet mild exercises that develop strength, endurance, and mobility.

Today, low-impact exercise for men includes a wide range of activities, from classic favorites like yoga and Pilates to cutting-edge routines like water aerobics and indoor rock climbing. These exercises have various advantages, including a lower chance of injury, better joint health, higher flexibility, and increased energy levels.

Furthermore, the accessibility of low-impact training has made it appealing to men of all ages and fitness levels. Whether recuperating from an accident, managing chronic diseases such as arthritis, or simply looking for a softer alternative to high-intensity exercises, men may discover a low-impact fitness plan that meets their requirements and goals.

Low-impact exercise for men dates back to ancient methods that emphasized mobility, balance, and flexibility. This notion has expanded over time to encompass a wide range of exercise activities that enhance health, energy, and longevity.

By adopting low-impact training, men may reach their fitness objectives safely and sustainably, assuring a lifetime of health and vitality.

# *What is Low Impact Exercise*

Low-impact exercise refers to physical activities that are easy on the joints and bones, making them appropriate for people of all fitness levels, including males.

These workouts reduce stress on the body while also giving several health advantages. Low-impact workouts are especially good for men who are recuperating from injuries, have joint problems, or simply want a less strenuous fitness regimen.

Low-impact workouts are known for their potential to lessen the risk of injury. Unlike high-impact sports like sprinting or leaping, which place a lot of strain on the joints, low-impact exercises are meant to be easier on the body.

This makes them perfect for guys who may already have joint difficulties or want to avoid injuries while remaining active.

Men's low-impact workouts include walking, swimming, cycling, and utilizing elliptical machines. These exercises allow for smooth, fluid motions without the jarring effect associated with more strenuous kinds of exercise.

Low-Impact workouts are easily adaptable to individual fitness levels and goals, making them accessible to a diverse spectrum of men, regardless of their present physical condition.

Low-impact activities not only reduce the danger of injury but also provide several health advantages. They can boost cardiovascular health, build muscle, and help you maintain a healthy weight. Low-impact activities are a great way for guys to enhance their fitness without placing too much strain on their bodies.

Another benefit of low-impact activities is their variety. They may be done indoors or outdoors, alone or in groups, making them appropriate for guys with a variety of inclinations and lives.

There are several low-impact exercise choices available, ranging from a leisurely bike ride through the neighborhood to an organized water aerobics session.

Low-impact activities may also be readily included in a well-rounded training regimen. Men can combine them with other types of exercise, such as strength training or flexibility exercises, to create a complete workout regimen that covers all elements of physical health.

This comprehensive strategy can promote general health and well-being.

Low-impact exercise provides men with a safe, effective, and adaptable approach to keep active and healthy. Low-impact workouts are a good choice for men of all ages and abilities since they reduce the chance of injury while still delivering several health advantages.

Walking, swimming, cycling, or any other low-impact activity can be incorporated into a regular fitness regimen to promote long-term health and well-being.

## *Benefits of Low Impact Exercise*

Low-impact exercise has several benefits for men, including a softer yet more effective method to increase fitness, health, and general well-being.

Unlike high-impact activities, which put substantial strain on the joints and muscles, low-impact exercises are gentler on the body, making them appropriate for people of all ages and fitness levels. Let's look at the overall benefits of low-impact exercise designed exclusively for males.

**1. Joint Health:** One of the most significant benefits of low-impact exercise is its mild nature, which decreases the chance of joint strain and damage. Low-impact workouts such as swimming, cycling, and walking can help men increase joint mobility and flexibility without increasing pain or discomfort, particularly those who already have joint difficulties or disorders such as arthritis.

**2. *Cardiovascular Health:*** Low-impact activities help to improve cardiovascular health by raising heart rate and circulation. Activities such as brisk walking, elliptical training, and rowing machines can help strengthen the heart, lower blood pressure, and minimize the risk of heart attack and stroke.

**3. *Weight Management:*** Low-impact exercise is a good alternative for guys who want to maintain their weight or lose extra pounds. While low-impact exercises may not burn calories as quickly as high-intensity workouts, they can still help you lose weight by increasing your metabolism and aiding fat burning.

**4. *Muscle Strength and Tone:*** Contrary to common opinion, low-impact exercise does not just provide cardiovascular advantages.

Many low-impact activities include many muscle groups, which help to increase strength, endurance, and total muscular tone.

Strength training using resistance bands, bodyweight exercises, or weight machines can help men gain lean muscle mass and functional strength.

**5. Stress Reduction:** Physical activity, particularly low-impact exercise, has been found to lower stress and increase mood by producing endorphins, the body's natural feel-good chemicals.

Men who include low-impact activities in their daily routine may have lower levels of anxiety, sadness, and general stress, leading to improved mental health.

**6. Long-Term Sustainability:** One of the most significant advantages of low-impact exercise is its long-term viability. Unlike high-intensity workouts, which can lead to burnout or overuse problems, low-impact activities are softer on the body, allowing people to continue a steady fitness routine without experiencing undue strain or exhaustion.

Low-impact exercise has several benefits for males, including increased joint health and cardiovascular fitness, as well as weight control, muscular strength, stress reduction, and long-term sustainability.

Men may attain their fitness objectives while reducing the chance of injury and improving their general health and well-being by including low-impact exercises in their routine.

# Common Misconceptions about Low Impact Exercise

Low-impact exercise is often disregarded or undervalued, particularly by males who prefer high-intensity workouts. However, there are numerous myths about low-impact exercise for males that should be addressed. In this detailed guide, we will refute these myths and discuss the benefits and relevance of adopting low-impact workouts into men's fitness regimens.

**Low Impact Means Low Intensity:** One common misperception is that low impact equals low intensity. While low-impact workouts are softer on the joints, they may still deliver an excellent cardiovascular workout while also helping to increase strength and endurance.

Swimming, cycling, and elliptical exercise can raise the heart rate and increase general fitness while putting little strain on the joints.

Many men assume that low-impact activities are ineffective for growing muscular growth. However, combining strength training with low-impact exercises can still promote muscle growth and endurance.

Bodyweight exercises, tension bands, and lightweight dumbbells can be utilized to engage muscles without putting them under as much strain as high-impact sports.

Another common myth is that low-impact activities burn fewer calories than high-impact ones. While high-intensity workouts like sprinting or jumping rope burn calories faster, low-impact exercises can also help with weight reduction and calorie expenditure, especially when done for extended periods or paired with interval training strategies.

**Not Tough Enough:** Some men may consider low-impact activities as too simple or insufficiently tough to produce substantial effects. Low-impact exercises may, however, be adapted to individual fitness levels and goals by varying intensity, and volume, and integrating progressive overload. Increasing resistance, adjusting tempo, or attempting new exercises can help keep workouts interesting and prevent plateaus.

**Only for Rehabilitation or Injury Recovery:** While low-impact workouts are frequently suggested for people recuperating from injuries or managing chronic diseases, they have additional benefits.

Incorporating low-impact activities into your daily training program can help you avoid injuries by minimizing joint tension and improving movement mechanics. Furthermore, they may be used as active recovery sessions in between more strenuous exercises, allowing muscles to recuperate while remaining active.

Low-impact exercise is an important part of men's fitness regimens since it provides several advantages without the risks associated with high-impact exercises

Men may maximize their exercise regimens and reach their health and wellness objectives sustainably by dispelling some common myths and recognizing the variety and effectiveness of low-impact activities.

# Chapter 2: Getting Started with Low Impact Exercise

Low-impact workouts are a fantastic choice for guys who want to increase their fitness without placing too much strain on their joints or muscles.

Whether you're recuperating from an injury, coping with joint discomfort, or simply prefer a mild approach to training, including low-impact workouts into your regimen can provide various advantages.

In this complete guide, we'll look at numerous low-impact workouts designed exclusively for males, as well as recommendations on how to get started efficiently.

### *Understanding Low Impact Exercises:*

Low-impact workouts are ones that put less stress on the joints while yet offering a cardiovascular and strength-building workout. These exercises are softer on the body than high-impact sports such as jogging or jumping, making them excellent for people who have joint concerns or want to lower their risk of injury.

### *Types of Low-Impact Exercises for Men:*

Walking: Brisk walking is a basic yet effective low-impact workout that you may easily add to your regular schedule. Aim for at least 30 minutes of brisk walking most days of the week to boost cardiovascular health and burn calories.

Swimming is a full-body activity that improves cardiovascular health without placing strain on the joints. Swimming, whether laps in the pool or water aerobics programs, is a flexible and low-impact workout for men of all ages.

***Cycling:*** Whether done outside or on a stationary cycle, cycling is a low-impact activity that builds leg muscles and improves cardiovascular health. Adjust the resistance and intensity to match your fitness level and objectives.

***Elliptical Training:*** The elliptical machine offers a smooth, low-impact workout that works several muscle groups, such as the legs, arms, and core. It's a terrific choice for males wishing to increase their cardiovascular endurance and lower body strength.

Yoga combines mild stretching, strength training, and relaxation methods, making it an excellent low-impact workout for men looking to enhance flexibility, balance, and stress alleviation. Find beginner-friendly yoga courses or online lessons to get started.

***Getting started:***

Before starting any new fitness routine, consult with a healthcare practitioner, especially if you have any pre-existing health issues or injuries.

To avoid overexertion and injury, begin with short exercises and gradually increase the time and intensity.

Invest in appropriate gear and equipment to assist your low-impact workout program while reducing the chance of pain or injury.

Listen to your body and make the necessary modifications.

If you encounter pain or discomfort while exercising, stop immediately and consult a certified specialist.

Incorporating low-impact activities into your daily routine can help you improve your health, fitness, and quality of life.

Men may reap the advantages of regular exercise without risking injury or discomfort by engaging in activities that are mild on the joints while also boosting strength, cardiovascular fitness, and flexibility.

 So lace up your sneakers, go in the pool, or lay out your yoga mat and start reaping the benefits of low-impact exercise now!

# Assessing Your Fitness Level

A fitness evaluation is essential for assessing your present physical condition and developing an appropriate training regimen. Assessing fitness levels is critical for men, particularly those looking for low-impact activities, to guarantee safe and long-term improvement.

Low-impact workouts have various advantages, including a lower chance of injury and joint stress, making them appropriate for men of all ages and fitness levels. Let's start by measuring fitness levels and looking for low-impact workouts that are appropriate for males.

**Assessing fitness levels:**

Cardiovascular Endurance: Assess your capacity to maintain physical exercise over time. Assessments such as the 1-mile walk test and the step test can determine your cardiovascular fitness level without putting too much strain on your joints.

***Muscular Strength and Endurance:*** Use push-ups, squats, and planks to assess upper, lower, and core strength. Aim for a certain number of repetitions based on your age and fitness objectives.

Assess your flexibility with easy tests such as the sit-and-reach or shoulder flexibility test. Flexibility is essential for preserving mobility and avoiding injuries, especially as men age.

***Balance and Stability:*** Balance tests, such as the single-leg stand or balance beam walk, can reveal proprioception and stability difficulties. Improving balance is essential for avoiding falls and increasing overall athleticism.

**Low-impact Exercises for Men:**

*Walking:* Incorporate brisk walking into your daily routine to boost cardiovascular health and burn calories. Begin with shorter workouts and progressively increase pace and distance as your fitness improves.

Swimming is a great full-body workout that puts no strain on joints. It increases cardiovascular endurance, strength, and flexibility while being gentle on the body.

*Riding:* Whether on a stationary cycle or outside, riding is a low-impact workout that builds leg muscles and boosts cardiovascular health. Adjust the resistance settings to progressively raise the intensity.

Yoga improves flexibility, balance, and mental focus through a sequence of positions and regulated breathing techniques. It also promotes relaxation and stress reduction, which are necessary for general well-being.

Pilates: Pilates employs regulated movements to improve core strength, flexibility, and alignment. It improves posture, stability, and muscular tone without placing tension on the joints.

Tai Chi is an ancient Chinese technique that includes soft, flowing motions, deep breathing, and meditation. Tai Chi improves balance, coordination, and mental clarity, making it appropriate for men of any age.

Include these low-impact activities in your training program to promote general health and well-being while reducing the chance of injury.
Always listen to your body, advance cautiously, and seek advice from a fitness professional as required. You may start a rewarding road to a healthier, more active

lifestyle by analyzing your fitness level and selecting appropriate workouts.

# Setting Realistic Goals

Setting realistic objectives is critical for success, particularly when including low-impact activities into a man's regimen. Setting attainable goals allows people to stay motivated, measure their progress, and avoid burnout or injury. Here's a thorough guide on creating realistic objectives for low-impact activities geared toward men:

Begin by assessing your current fitness level. Consider age, weight, general health, and any current injuries or diseases. This examination will assist in establishing a starting point and setting realistic goals.

**speak with a practitioner:** Before beginning any workout program, you should speak with a healthcare practitioner or trained trainer. They may provide tailored suggestions based on your health and fitness objectives, assuring safety and efficacy.

Set specific goals. Set clear and defined goals for your low-impact workout regimen. Rather than setting general goals like "get in shape," strive for specific results such as increased flexibility, endurance, or stress reduction.

***Consider Low-Impact Workouts:*** Choose workouts that are easy on the joints and muscles, such as swimming, walking, cycling, yoga, or tai chi. These activities offer cardiovascular advantages without placing too much effort on the body.

***Start Slowly and Progress Gradually:*** Resist the urge to push too hard too quickly. Begin with moderate workout durations and intensities, gradually increasing as your fitness improves. This strategy reduces the danger of harm while allowing for long-term improvement.

***Set Realistic Timeframes:*** Be realistic about how long it will take to attain your goals. Significant fitness transformations need time and perseverance, just as Rome was not created overnight. Determine short and long-term objectives with realistic timelines depending on your current fitness level and lifestyle commitments.

Track your exercises, progress, and successes. This can be accomplished with an exercise diary, a fitness app, or a wearable fitness tracker. Monitoring your progress can help you stay motivated and find areas for growth.

***Adjust as needed:*** Be adaptable and open to changing your goals as necessary. Life events, accidents, or shifts in priorities may need changes to your workout regimen. Adaptability is essential for maintaining a long-term commitment to exercise.

***Milestones:*** Recognize and celebrate significant achievements along the road. Recognizing accomplishments, whether it's meeting a weight reduction goal, mastering a new yoga posture, or increasing endurance, promotes motivation and reinforces healthy habits.

***Focus on total Well-being:*** Keep in mind that fitness is only one component of total well-being. Prioritize overall health by combining balanced eating, proper sleep, stress management skills, and regular medical check-ups into your daily routine.

Setting realistic objectives for low-impact workouts allows men to reap the advantages of increased fitness and well-being while reducing the chance of injury or burnout. A healthy lifestyle is achievable and sustainable with patience, persistence, and drive.

## *Creating a Personalized Low Impact Exercise Plan*

When it comes to fitness, it's critical to personalize your workout regimen to your own needs and tastes.

For men looking for a low-impact workout routine, various choices can assist increase strength, flexibility, and cardiovascular health without placing excessive strain on the joints. Here's a detailed approach to developing a tailored low-impact workout program:

Before starting an exercise regimen, it's important to evaluate your present fitness level. This might help you decide where to start and create achievable goals. Consider your general health, any current injuries or ailments, and your workout history.

Before starting a new fitness routine, seek advice from a healthcare practitioner if you have any underlying health issues or injuries. They can provide tailored suggestions and guarantee that you're participating in safe and successful activities.

***Choose Low-Impact Exercises:*** These exercises are mild on joints and provide an efficient workout. Walking, cycling, swimming, yoga, tai chi, and elliptical machines are a few examples. Including a range of workouts might help you avoid boredom and target different muscle regions.

Strength exercise helps grow muscle mass, boost metabolism, and improve overall strength and endurance.

To minimize severe joint stress, use activities that use body weight, resistance bands, or light dumbbells. Aim to add strength training exercises at least two to three times per week, focusing on key muscular groups such as the chest, back, legs, and core.

***Prioritize Flexibility and Balance:*** A well-rounded fitness regimen requires flexibility and balance, especially for older men.

Stretching techniques like yoga or Pilates can help increase flexibility and range of motion. Practice balance exercises like single-leg stand or stability ball exercises to improve proprioception and lower your chance of falling.

As your fitness increases, progressively raise the intensity of your workouts to keep your body challenged. This might include increasing the time or intensity of your workouts, using resistance, or attempting more sophisticated versions.

Listen to your body and don't push too hard, especially if you're new to exercising or recuperating from an injury.

Adjust your workout routine based on your body's response. If you are experiencing pain or discomfort, alter or discontinue the offending workouts and, if required, check with a healthcare practitioner.

Following these principles and adjusting your workout plan to your own goals and tastes will allow you to establish a tailored low-impact fitness program that supports men's overall health and well-being.

# *Chapter 3: Cardiovascular Low Impact Exercises*

Cardiovascular health is critical to overall well-being, particularly for men who want to retain their fitness and vigor. Low-impact workouts are a fantastic approach to enhance cardiovascular health without placing too much strain on the joints, making them suitable for men of all ages and fitness levels.

Let's look at some thorough and detailed low-impact cardiovascular workouts designed exclusively for men:

Walking is one of the easiest and effective low-impact cardiovascular workouts, but while is often overlooked. To get your heart pounding and boost circulation, aim for at least 30 minutes of exercise every day, whether it's a brisk stroll outside or on a treadmill.

Cycling: Whether stationary or outdoor, cycling is a fantastic cardiovascular activity that is easy on the joints. Adjust the resistance to challenge yourself and progressively build endurance over time.

Swimming is a full-body workout that is very mild on the joints. It works for numerous muscle groups and provides a terrific cardiovascular exercise. To keep things fresh, try various strokes such as freestyle, breaststroke, and backstroke.

***Elliptical Training:*** The elliptical machine is a low-impact alternative to running that yet gives good cardiovascular exercise. It simulates the motion of walking or running without causing jarring effects on the knees and hips.

Rowing machines offer a low-impact, full-body workout that develops the cardiovascular system and targets muscles in the arms, back, and legs. To push yourself, maintain excellent form while progressively increasing resistance.

Look for aerobics sessions that focus on low-impact routines. These programs often include rhythmic motions that raise the heart rate while minimizing joint stress.

*Stair Climbing:* Use stair-stepper machines or find a set of steps to climb for a difficult but low-impact cardiovascular workout. Begin with a reasonable number of repetitions and progressively raise the intensity as your fitness increases.

*Tai Chi:* This ancient Chinese martial art mixes gentle, flowing motions with deep breathing exercises. Tai Chi enhances cardiovascular health, balance, and flexibility while also encouraging relaxation and stress reduction.

Incorporating these low-impact cardiovascular workouts into your program will help men improve their heart health, endurance, and weight management while avoiding injury or joint strain.

Consistency is essential, so schedule frequent exercise sessions to gain the full advantages of better cardiovascular health. Always contact with a healthcare expert before beginning any new fitness routine, especially if you have pre-existing health concerns.

## *Walking - The Ultimate Low Impact Cardio*

Walking is often regarded as the best low-impact aerobic exercise for men, providing several health advantages while placing no pressure on the joints.

Whether you're a fitness fanatic or just starting on your path to a better lifestyle, adding walking into your daily routine may be revolutionary. Let's look at the several benefits and insights into walking as a low-impact fitness alternative for guys.

First and foremost, walking is easy on the joints, making it suitable for men of all ages and fitness levels. Walking, as opposed to high-impact exercises such as sprinting or leaping, which can stress the joints and cause problems over time, provides a smooth and natural range of motion, lowering the risk of joint discomfort and inflammation.

Walking is a versatile workout that can be readily included in everyday routines. Whether it's a brisk walk during your lunch break, a stroll in the evening, or incorporating walking into your commute by taking stairs instead of elevators, there are endless ways to incorporate walking into your routine that don't require specialized equipment or dedicated gym time.

Walking has several advantages, including its ability to improve cardiovascular health. Regular walking can help men reduce their risk of heart disease, stroke, and hypertension. Walking at a moderate speed for 30 minutes each day can considerably enhance heart health by boosting circulation, lowering blood pressure, and decreasing LDL cholesterol levels.

Walking also has several mental health advantages. According to research, daily walking can help reduce symptoms of sadness and anxiety, raise mood, and improve general cognitive performance.

Walking's rhythmic action, along with exposure to the outdoors and fresh air, may have a relaxing impact on the mind, making it a good stress-relief exercise for men who must balance work and family life.

Walking is a very versatile activity that may be adjusted to specific fitness objectives. Walking may be tailored to your personal goals, whether you want to lose weight, enhance your endurance, or simply maintain an active lifestyle.

By varying the duration, intensity, and terrain of your walks, you may push your body and work toward your fitness objectives over time.

Walking stands out as the best low-impact cardio activity for males, providing several health advantages without putting excessive strain on the body.

Walking promotes joint health and cardiovascular fitness while also improving emotional well-being and weight control. Walking daily can provide you with years of increased health and vigor.

## *Swimming - Gentle on Joints, Effective for Cardio*

Swimming is a low-impact workout that has several benefits, especially for men who want to maintain cardiovascular health while being easy on their joints.

This complete workout works for numerous muscular groups at once, making it an efficient approach to building strength, endurance, and general fitness without placing too much strain on the body.

One of the key benefits of swimming is its low stress on the joints. Swimming, unlike high-impact workouts like jogging or weightlifting, which can cause joint pain and discomfort over time, allows people to exercise without putting too much strain on their joints. This makes it an excellent choice for guys who already have joint problems or want to avoid developing them in the future.

Swimming is a great cardiovascular workout. Swimmers can increase their heart rate and cardiovascular endurance by continually swimming against the resistance of the water.

Whether swimming laps in the pool or swimming in open water, this aerobic activity strengthens the heart and lungs, lowering the risk of heart disease, stroke, and other cardiovascular diseases.

Swimming, in addition to its cardiovascular advantages, is a full-body workout that works for many different muscle groups. Swimming strokes exercise almost every muscle in the body, including the arms, shoulders, core, and legs.

This total muscle involvement not only increases strength but also flexibility and coordination, resulting in improved overall physical performance.

Swimming provides a unique combination of resistance and buoyancy. The water offers natural resistance, making the muscles work harder with each stroke.

Resistance exercise increases muscular growth and tones the body, resulting in a leaner, more defined physique. At the same time, water's buoyancy minimizes the impact on joints, allowing people to exercise more easily and comfortably.

Swimming can be an excellent weight-management technique for males. Swimming regularly can help people reach and maintain a healthy weight since aerobic exercises burn more calories. Swimming also improves metabolism, which leads to increased calorie expenditure long after the activity is completed.

Finally, swimming has significant mental health advantages. Swimming strokes are rhythmic, and the calming characteristics of water can encourage relaxation and lower stress levels.

Many swimmers discover that the contemplative component of swimming gives a welcome respite from the stresses of everyday life, resulting in increased mood and overall well-being.

Swimming is a good low-impact workout for men wanting to enhance cardiovascular health, gain strength, and maintain overall fitness. Its gentle nature makes yoga appropriate for people of all ages and fitness levels, and its many advantages extend beyond physical health to mental and emotional well-being.

Swimming as part of a regular fitness plan can result in considerable health and quality of life benefits.

## *Cycling - Building Endurance Without Strain*

Cycling is a fantastic low-impact workout for guys looking to increase endurance without putting too much effort on their bodies.

Cycling, whether done outdoors or on stationary cycles, has several benefits for cardiovascular health, muscle strength, and overall well-being. Let's look at how cycling may help guys build endurance effectively and safely.

One of the primary benefits of cycling is its low-impact nature. Cycling, unlike high-impact exercises like running or leaping, puts less stress on the joints, making it suitable for men who have joint problems or are recuperating from injuries.

This makes it a long-term workout choice for increasing endurance while avoiding injury or worsening pre-existing problems.

Cycling provides an excellent cardiovascular workout, boosting the heart and lungs while increasing circulation. Regular cycling helps to lower blood pressure, lessen the risk of heart disease, and increase overall cardiovascular fitness.

Men can enhance their endurance levels without stressing their hearts by gradually increasing the length and intensity of their rides.

Cycling works many muscular groups, including the quadriceps, hamstrings, calves, and glutes. As men pedal, these muscles combine to move the bike ahead, eventually increasing strength and endurance.

Over time, frequent cycling workouts build muscular stamina, allowing men to cycle greater distances with less fatigue. This is especially useful for hobbies that require consistent effort, such as long-distance cycling or mountain riding.

***Weight Management:*** Cycling may be a very helpful technique for guys who want to lose weight or keep their weight stable. It is a calorie-burning exercise that boosts metabolic rate and aids in weight reduction.

Men who incorporate cycling into their training program can establish a calorie deficit, resulting in moderate but long-term weight loss. Cycling helps tone and shape leg muscles, resulting in a more defined body.

Cycling has several mental health benefits in addition to physical ones. Riding outside exposes males to fresh air, sunlight, and picturesque sights, which can improve mood and reduce stress. The repetitive action of cycling encourages relaxation and awareness, giving a pleasant break from the stresses of everyday life. Cycling may also be a social sport, allowing men to meet others who share their enthusiasm for bicycling.

Cycling is an excellent choice for guys looking to increase endurance without exertion. Its low-impact nature, cardiovascular advantages, muscle strengthening effects, weight-management possibilities, and favorable influence on mental health make it an excellent workout choice.

Men who incorporate cycling into their training routine may increase their endurance, improve their general health, and enjoy the exciting freedom of the open road or the invigorating challenge of indoor cycling courses.

# *Chapter 4: Strength Training with Low Impact*

Strength training with low-impact exercises provides men with a varied and efficient technique to gain muscle, enhance general fitness, and reduce stress on joints and connective tissues.

These workouts emphasize regulated motions and lower resistance, reducing strain on the body while yet giving considerable benefits. Here's a complete summary of low-impact strength training for men:

**Advantages of Low-impact Strength Training:**

**Reduced chance of injury:** Low-impact workouts place less strain on joints, making them excellent for men who have joint problems or are recuperating from injuries. Low-impact strength training can assist in maintaining joint health and avoid problems such as osteoarthritis by encouraging good alignment and controlled motions.

***Enhanced muscular strength and endurance:***

Despite the reduced impact, these workouts stimulate muscle growth and enhance strength, allowing men to reach their fitness objectives while avoiding injury.
Key exercises:

***Bodyweight exercises:*** Push-ups, squats, lunges, and planks are all good bodyweight exercises that may be tailored to individual fitness levels.
Resistance band exercises: Resistance bands have adjustable resistance levels and may target many muscle areas, giving a

demanding workout without using heavy weights.

**Dumbbell exercises:** Using lighter dumbbells with perfect technique may efficiently target particular muscle groups while putting less load on joints.

**Stability ball exercises:** Including stability balls in strength training routines can help increase balance, stability, and core strength while having little impact on joints. Sample Low Impact Strength Training Routine:

**Warm-up:** Perform five to ten minutes of modest aerobic exercise to stimulate blood flow and prepare the muscles for activities. Bodyweight circuit: Do a circuit of bodyweight exercises such as push-ups, squats, lunges, and planks, performing 10-15 repetitions of each with a little break in between sets.

***Resistance band workouts:*** Incorporate resistance band exercises such as bicep curls, shoulder presses, and rows, with 2-3 sets of 12-15 repetitions for each exercise.

Dumbbell workouts include chest presses, overhead tricep extensions, and lateral lifts, with a focus on appropriate technique and control.

Finish with stability ball exercises, such as crunches, hamstring curls, and pelvic lifts, to target core muscles and enhance stability.
Cool down and stretching:

Finish the workout with five to ten minutes of gentle aerobic activity to gradually reduce your heart rate and encourage recovery.
Finish with stretching exercises that target main muscle groups to increase flexibility and minimize muscular pain.

Incorporating low-impact strength training into a fitness regimen can help men accomplish their fitness goals while reducing injury risk and improving long-term joint health. Men can increase their overall fitness by concentrating on controlled movements, excellent technique, and lighter resistance.

# Bodyweight Exercises for Strength and Tone

Bodyweight exercises are a popular way to increase strength and tone muscles without the need for expensive equipment or heavy weights.

They are not only effective but also low-impact, making them appropriate for men of all ages and levels of fitness. Here's a complete introduction to some of the greatest bodyweight workouts for strength and tone, with an emphasis on low-impact options:

**Push-ups:** A basic workout that works the chest, shoulders, and triceps. To do a push-up, begin in a plank posture with your hands shoulder-width apart, then lower your body until your chest almost touches the ground before pushing back up to the starting position.

Bodyweight squats help to strengthen your lower body. Stand with your feet shoulder-width apart, then lower your body as if sitting back in a chair, keeping your knees behind your toes.

To return to the beginning position, push through your heels.

Lunges help to improve balance and leg strength.

Take a step forward with one leg, then lower yourself until both knees are bent at a 90-degree angle.

Push back up to the starting position, then repeat with the other leg.

**Planks:** Use planks to strengthen your core muscles. Begin in a push-up posture, but keep your forearms on the ground.

Hold your body in a straight line from head to heels, using your core muscles throughout.

Glute bridges are exercises that target your glutes and hamstrings.

With feet flat on the ground, knees bent lie on your back.

 Lift your hips to the ceiling, squeezing your glutes at the peak, then drop back down and repeat.

Pull-ups and chin-ups will help you work your back, biceps, and forearm muscles.

Grip a bar with hands slightly wider than shoulder-width apart (pull-ups) or closer together with palms facing you (chin-ups), then lift your body until your chin clears the bar, then drop and repeat.

***Tricep Dips:*** Tricep dips are an exercise that works the triceps. Sit on the edge of a chair or bench, clutching it with your hands.

Slide your hips off the edge, bend your elbows to lower your body until your arms create a 90-degree angle, and push back up to the starting position.

Incorporating these low-impact bodyweight exercises into your regimen will help you gain strength, muscular tone, and general fitness without placing too much strain on your joints.

Aim to do each exercise with perfect form, gradually increasing repetitions or difficulty as you go.

With determination and consistency, you may attain your strength and tone objectives utilizing only your body weight.

## Resistance Band Workouts - Versatile and Joint-Friendly

In a fitness scene dominated by heavy weights and high-impact exercises, resistance band workouts provide a welcome alternative, especially for men looking for low-impact yet effective training choices.

These elastic bands, which are sometimes disregarded in favor of typical gym equipment, offer a flexible and joint-friendly approach to strength training and recovery.

Let's look at the advantages and variety of resistance band workouts designed exclusively for guys who want to improve their joint health and general well-being.

**1. Joint-Friendly Strength Training:** One of the key benefits of resistance band workouts is their ability to deliver resistance while placing minimal strain on the joints. Resistance bands are a mild but efficient technique to improve strength and muscle mass for guys who have joint concerns or just want to reduce wear and tear.

**2. *Flexibility for Total-Body Workouts:*** Resistance bands may target every major muscle group in the body, from the upper to the lower and the core. Whether doing bicep curls, chest presses, squats, or lunges, these bands maintain continuous tension throughout the full range of motion, resulting in a complete exercise that pushes muscles from all angles.

**3. *Adjustable Resistance Levels:*** One of the most important aspects of resistance bands is the ability to simply modify resistance levels. Men may adapt the intensity of their exercises to their fitness levels and goals by simply increasing the tension of the bands or utilizing numerous bands at the same time. Resistance bands may be used by people of all fitness levels, from novices to expert athletes, because of their scalability.

**4. Portable and Convenient:** Resistance bands, unlike bulkier gym equipment, are lightweight, portable, and take up little room, making them great for home workouts or travel. Men may easily pack a couple of bands in their gym bag or luggage to ensure they never miss a workout, whether at home, at work, or on the go.

**5. Improved Stability and Balance:** Resistance band workouts frequently work stabilizer muscles, which are critical for maintaining balance and avoiding injuries. Men may enhance their general balance and coordination by including workouts that test stability, such as single-leg squats or standing rows, which will result in greater performance in sports and daily activities.

### 6. Rehabilitation and Injury Prevention:

For males healing from injuries or suffering from chronic pain, resistance bands may be quite useful for rehabilitation and injury prevention.
Resistance band workouts are regulated and low-impact, allowing people to develop muscles, improve flexibility, and increase joint stability without worsening pre-existing ailments.

Resistance band workouts for men provide a diverse, joint-friendly, and effective alternative to standard strength training approaches.

Resistance bands are a must-have for any low-impact training regimen since they provide adjustable resistance, target different muscle areas, and enhance joint health.

By including these flexible tools in their training routine, men may reach their strength and wellness objectives while reducing the chance of injury and increasing overall health and lifespan.

## *Incorporating Yoga for Strength and Flexibility*

Yoga, which is traditionally linked with flexibility and relaxation, is becoming more well-recognized for its benefits in developing strength and overall fitness, making it a great low-impact workout alternative for males.

Men who include yoga in their workout regimens can improve their physical performance, avoid injuries, and increase mental health.

Yoga not only focuses on stretching but also incorporates strength-building poses that target specific muscle areas. Plank, Chaturanga, and Warrior routines target the core, arms, shoulders, and legs, promoting functional strength. These postures frequently demand holding positions for a lengthy amount of time, which tests muscles in ways that standard weightlifting does not. In addition, many yoga positions require balance, which develops stabilizing muscles and improves general body control.

Improving flexibility is critical for preserving joint health and reducing injuries, especially in older men. Yoga increases flexibility by gradually stretching and extending muscles, tendons, and ligaments.

Downward Facing Dog, Forward Fold, and Pigeon position stretch hamstrings, hips, and lower back. Regular practice progressively enhances the range of motion, making ordinary activities simpler and more pleasant while decreasing the likelihood of strains and sprains.

Yoga is a low-impact exercise that can benefit men of all ages and fitness levels, especially those recuperating from injuries or experiencing joint concerns. Unlike high-impact exercises such as jogging or weightlifting, which can stress the joints and cause wear and tear over time, yoga puts less demand on the body while giving an efficient workout. This makes it an excellent choice for preserving fitness and mobility while avoiding worsening current issues.

Yoga provides both physical and mental health advantages, such as stress reduction, greater attention, and mood control.

The combination of breath practice (pranayama) and mindful movement helps to quiet the nervous system, promote relaxation, and alleviate the consequences of chronic stress. Regular yoga practice has been related to decreased anxiety and sadness, making it an effective tool for general well-being.

Yoga may be a great addition to any exercise program for guys looking to increase their strength, flexibility, and general health. Yoga, with its emphasis on functional movement, low-impact nature, and mental health benefits, provides a complete approach to fitness that addresses both physical and emotional wellness.

Yoga, whether performed alone or in conjunction with other types of exercise, offers men of all ages a diverse and accessible way to achieve and maintain maximum health and fitness.

# Chapter 5: Flexibility and Mobility Exercises

Flexibility and mobility are essential components of total fitness, especially for men seeking to maintain peak health and performance.

Incorporating low-impact workouts into your program can increase joint range of motion, lower your risk of injury, and boost athletic performance. Below is a thorough introduction to flexibility and mobility exercises designed exclusively for guys.

**1. Begin with active stretching**: movements to warm up the muscles and enhance blood flow. These movements include arm circles, leg swings, and torso twists. Dynamic stretching prepares the body for action and helps to avoid damage during training.

**2. Foam Rolling:** Foam rolling is a useful practice for reducing muscular tension and increasing mobility. Concentrate on regions prone to tension, such as the calves, quadriceps, and hamstring. Spend 1-2 minutes rolling each muscle group.

**3. Yoga and Pilates:** Both yoga and Pilates focus on flexibility, mobility, and core strength. Include poses and motions that target specific regions of tension, such as a downward dog for hamstrings and a child's pose for lower back relief. These routines also encourage relaxation and stress reduction.

**4. Resistance Band Exercises:** Resistance bands are a flexible tool for increasing flexibility and movement. Exercises for shoulder mobility include band pull-aparts, band walks for hip stability, and band hamstring stretches for greater flexibility.

**5. *Tai Chi:*** Tai Chi is a low-impact martial art that emphasizes slow, controlled movement and deep breathing. Tai Chi may help you improve your balance, coordination, and joint mobility, as well as relax and clear your mind.

**6. *Swimming:*** Swimming is a great low-impact workout that works the entire body and provides mild resistance. It enhances flexibility, muscle strength, and cardiovascular health while minimizing joint stress.

**7. *Mobility Drills:*** Use particular mobility drills to target regions of stiffness or limited range of motion. Examples include broomstick-assisted shoulder dislocations, hip circles, and ankle rotations. These workouts assist in lubricating joints and improve movement patterns.

**8. *Stretching program:*** Create a regular stretching program that targets key muscular areas such as the hamstrings, quadriceps, calves, chest, shoulders, and back. Hold each stretch for 20-30 seconds, then repeat 2-3 times. Breathe deeply and relax into the stretch.

Finally, men of all ages and fitness levels should incorporate flexibility and mobility exercises into their workout routines.

Men who include dynamic stretching, foam rolling, yoga, resistance bands, Tai Chi, swimming, mobility exercises, and regular stretching practice can increase joint range of motion, minimize injury risk, and improve overall health and performance.

Begin adding these workouts into your daily regimen today to get the advantages firsthand.

## *Stretching for Improved Range of Motion*

Stretching is an essential part of any workout practice, providing several advantages such as increased flexibility, range of motion, and injury prevention. Stretching exercises can be very useful for males, especially when they focus on low-impact, joint-friendly movements.

Let's go into the specifics of stretching for greater range of motion, with a focus on males looking for low-impact choices.

Stretching helps maintain optimal muscle function and joint health. Stretching reduces stress and stiffness by lengthening muscles and tendons, improving flexibility and range of motion. Stretching can help avoid muscular imbalances, minimize the chance of injury, and increase general physical well-being in males, particularly those who engage in weightlifting or high-intensity activities.

**Key Low-Impact Stretching Exercises For Men:**

**Hamstring Stretch:** Sit on the floor with one leg extended and the other bent, with the foot on the inner thigh. Reach towards the outstretched foot while maintaining your back straight. Hold for 20-30 seconds then swap sides.

**Quadriceps Stretch:** Stand up straight, holding onto a wall or chair for balance if necessary. Grab one ankle and slowly move it toward the buttocks while maintaining the knees close together.

Repeat on the opposite side after holding for 20 to 40 seconds

***Calf Stretch:*** Stand facing a wall, one foot forward and the other back, both feet flat on the floor. Lean forward while maintaining the rear leg straight until you feel a stretch in your calf muscle. Hold for 20-30 seconds then swap sides.

Kneel on one knee and place the other foot flat on the ground in front of you, forming a 90-degree angle with your knee. Gently lean forward while maintaining your back straight, until you feel a stretch at the front of your hip. Hold for 20-30 seconds then swap sides.

***Shoulder Stretch:*** Stand tall and reach one arm across the body, gently pressing the opposite hand on the chest until you feel a stretch in your shoulder.

Repeat on the opposite side after holding for 20 to 40 seconds

To maximize the advantages of stretching, men should add it into their training program 2-3 times per week. Stretching should be done after a warm-up or workout, when the muscles are warm and flexible. To optimize efficacy, hold each stretch for 20-30 seconds while focusing on deep breathing and relaxation.

stretching is an essential component of any workout program for men looking to increase their flexibility, range of motion, and overall physical performance. Men who incorporate these low-impact stretching exercises into their routine may improve their mobility, avoid injuries, and maximize their health and fitness levels in the long run.

# Tai Chi - Flowing Movements for Balance and Flexibility

Tai Chi, an ancient Chinese martial art, has grown in popularity across the world as a low-impact workout with various advantages, particularly for men who want to enhance their balance, flexibility, and general health.

Its soft, flowing motions make yoga suitable for people of all ages and fitness levels, while the contemplative component promotes mental clarity and stress reduction.

**1. *Low-Impact Exercise:*** Tai Chi consists of slow, methodical motions that place less stress on the joints, making it suitable for men looking for a low-impact type of exercise. Unlike high-impact exercises such as jogging or weightlifting, Tai Chi allows people to improve their bodies while avoiding injury or strain.

**2. *Improved Balance:*** One of the primary advantages of Tai Chi is its ability to improve balance and stability. Practitioners get a heightened sense of balance through a sequence of controlled motions and shifting of body weight, lowering their risk of falls and accidents, especially as they age.

**3. *Flexibility and Joint Health:*** Tai Chi's gentle stretches and rotations promote flexibility and joint health. Regular practice can result in an enhanced range of motion, making everyday tasks easier and more pleasant for men, especially those with stiff or tight muscles.

**4. *Stress Reduction:*** In addition to its physical advantages, Tai Chi is well-known for its ability to reduce stress. The slow, rhythmic motions, along with deep breathing and concentrated concentration, aid in relaxation and mental clarity. This is especially useful for guys struggling with work-related stress or other life stresses.

**5. *Mind-Body Connection:*** Tai Chi is frequently referred to as a movement meditation that emphasizes the relationship between the mind and body. Practitioners develop increased awareness and mindfulness by focusing on the present moment and the sensations in their bodies, resulting in a sense of inner peace and harmony.

**6. *Cardiovascular Health:*** Although Tai Chi is not a high-intensity aerobic exercise, studies have shown that frequent practice can benefit cardiovascular health. The mild motions improve blood flow and circulation, lowering blood pressure and decreasing the risk of heart disease.

**7. *Social Engagement:*** Tai Chi sessions allow guys to mingle and connect with people who have similar health and well-being goals. The friendly environment fosters friendship and motivation, improving the whole experience of Tai Chi.

Tai Chi is a comprehensive approach to health and fitness that incorporates physical exercise, mental relaxation, and spiritual well-being. Its flowing motions, mild nature, and ease of use make it an excellent choice for men looking to enhance their balance, flexibility, and general quality of life through a low-impact training regimen.

## *Pilates - Core Strengthening for Better Posture and Alignment*

Maintaining excellent posture and alignment is critical for general health and well-being, especially for men who must deal with the demands of employment, physical activity, and aging.

Core strengthening exercises are essential for establishing and maintaining good posture and alignment because they target the muscles that support the spine and pelvis. Here's a whole guide to low-impact core workouts particularly designed for men:

### 1. Plank variations:

***Standard Plank:*** Start in a push-up posture, with your hands precisely under your shoulders and your body in a straight line from head to heels. Hold for 30 seconds to a minute, focusing on your core muscles.

**Side Plank:** Lie on your side, elbows just behind your shoulders, legs stacked.

 Lift your hips until your body is in a straight line from head to heels.

 Hold for 30 seconds on both sides.

**Forearm Plank:** Like a conventional plank, but with your forearms on the ground.

Maintain a straight line from head to heels and hold for 30 seconds to 1 minute.

## 2. Birddog:

Beggin on your hands and knees, placing your wrists precisely under your shoulders and your knees beneath your hips.

Extend your right arm forward and your left leg back while keeping your hips level and your spine neutral.

Hold for a few seconds before returning to the start position and switching sides.

Repeat 10–15 times on each side.

### 3. Deadbug:

Lie on your back, arms stretched to the ceiling, knees bent at a 90-degree angle.

Slowly drop your right arm and left leg to the ground while maintaining your lower back flat on the floor.

Repeat on the opposite side after returning to your starting position

Aim for 10-15 repetitions per side.

### 4. Pelvic tilts.

With feet flat on the floor and legs bent,pay on your back

Engage your core muscles and tilt your pelvis upward, forcing your lower back into the ground.

Hold for a few seconds and then release. Repeat for 10-15 repetitions.

### 5. Bridge:

With feet flat on the floor and legs bent,pay on your back

Lift your hips to the ceiling, clenching your glutes and activating your core.

Hold for a few seconds at the peak before lowering back down. Aim for 10–15 repetitions.

Including these low-impact core strengthening exercises in your workout program will help you improve your posture, alignment, and general stability. Remember to maintain appropriate form and technique while progressively increasing the intensity and length as you gain strength. Consistency is crucial, so incorporate these exercises into your training program at least 2-3 times each week for best results.

# *Chapter 6: Low Impact Exercises for Joint Health*

Maintaining joint health is critical for men of all ages, especially as they deal with hectic schedules, demanding occupations, and numerous physical activities.

Low-impact workouts may transform a training regimen by providing a mild yet effective technique to build muscles, enhance flexibility, and boost general joint health without generating unneeded strain. Let's look at some unusual and exciting low-impact workouts designed for men:

**Paddleboarding:** Take to the water for a great low-impact exercise that strengthens core muscles, improves balance, and increases joint stability. Paddleboarding, whether on a tranquil lake or surfing mild waves at the beach, gives you a full-body workout while reducing joint tension.

Furthermore, the quiet surroundings provide a welcome respite from the hurry and bustle of daily life.

***Trail Walking:*** Get outside and hit the trails for a low-impact walking workout that helps both your body and mind. Trail walking allows men to immerse themselves in nature while strengthening leg muscles, increasing cardiovascular health, and reducing joint stiffness.

With diverse terrain and scenery, each walk becomes an adventure, making it an enjoyable and refreshing form of exercise.

***Rowing Machine Workouts:*** Rowing machines provide a low-impact, full-body workout that works for numerous muscle groups at once. Men can enjoy rowing's rhythmic action, which strengthens the arms, back, and legs while giving a great cardiovascular workout. Rowing machine training, whether at home or the gym, may be tailored to specific fitness levels and objectives.

Pilates is a low-impact workout regimen that focuses on developing core strength, flexibility, and body awareness.

Pilates workouts comprise regulated motions done on a mat or with specialist equipment, which helps men create long, lean muscles and improve posture while minimizing joint stress.

Pilates, with its emphasis on exact technique and breath control, provides a unique approach to exercise that improves general well-being.

Rock climbing is a fascinating low-impact activity that tests strength, endurance, and problem-solving abilities. Indoor climbing gyms provide men with a safe and supervised place to study and practice climbing methods while increasing upper body and grip strength. Rock climbing works muscles all throughout the body without subjecting the joints to high-impact pressures, making it a thrilling but joint-friendly sport.

Qi Gong is an ancient Chinese practice that promotes balance, harmony, and energy in both the body and the mind.

Qi Gong is a set of gentle movements, breathing exercises, and meditation techniques used to increase the flow of Qi (life force) throughout the body. Men can benefit from better flexibility, less tension, and increased joint mobility by practicing Qi Gong daily, which provides a tranquil and contemplative approach to exercise.

Incorporating these new and innovative low-impact activities into a weekly regimen will help men prioritize joint health while also providing different and gratifying workout experiences. By embracing variation and listening to their bodies, men may discover new methods to stay active, energetic, and resilient for many years.

## Aquatic Therapy - Relieving Joint Pain with Water Workouts

Aquatic therapy, often known as water therapy or hydrotherapy, is a therapeutic method that uses the qualities of water to promote healing and well-being.

This type of treatment is especially good for those who have joint pain since it provides a low-impact workout setting that can help them feel better and move more freely. For men with joint problems, water treatment provides a complete and successful way to control discomfort while remaining active.

**Low-impact exercises for men:**

Men, particularly those having joint discomfort or recovering from injuries, frequently seek workout choices that are mild on the body while yet improving strength and flexibility. Traditional kinds of exercise, such as jogging or weightlifting, can aggravate joint pain and lead to more injury. Aquatic treatment, on the other hand, provides a low-impact setting that decreases joint tension while yet allowing for the complete range of motion.

**Comprehensive Benefits of Aquatic Therapy:**

*Reduced Joint Stress:* Water buoyancy mitigates the effects of gravity on the body, reducing the strain on joints during activity. This enables males with joint discomfort to participate in activities that would be too difficult on land, such as walking or light stretching, without incurring further strain.

*Improved Range of Motion:* Water resistance provides a natural kind of resistance training that strengthens muscles and increases joint flexibility. Men who engage in water treatment can progressively expand their range of motion without risking harm, resulting in better mobility over time.

*Pain Management:* The therapeutic warmth of water soothes tight muscles and relieves joint pain. Furthermore, the mild pressure of water helps reduce inflammation and swelling, bringing comfort to males suffering from arthritis or tendonitis.

*Improved Cardiovascular Health:* Aquatic sports, such as swimming or water aerobics, can boost cardiovascular endurance without placing a load on joints. Men can engage in aerobic exercises that increase heart rate and improve overall fitness while lowering their risk of impact-related injuries.

*Improved Balance and Coordination:* The unstable nature of water forces the body to use stabilizing muscles, resulting in better balance and coordination. This is especially useful for elderly males and those recuperating from injuries who are in danger of falling.

Aquatic treatment provides men with a complete and efficient way to relieve joint discomfort and improve general fitness.

Despite joint difficulties, water therapy allows men to be active and retain a good quality of life by offering a low-impact workout setting that decreases joint stress while developing strength, flexibility, and cardiovascular health.

Whether used alone or in combination with other therapeutic approaches, water therapy has enormous promise for men looking for joint pain alleviation and a route to better health.

## *Balance Exercises to Support Joint Stability*

Achieving and maintaining joint stability is critical for general health and mobility, especially for men who wish to stay active and avoid injury.

Low-impact balancing exercises may significantly improve your workout regimen. Here's a look at some new and innovative workouts designed to improve joint stability:

**1. *Water Workouts:*** Practice balancing exercises in the pool. Water offers resistance without placing strain on your joints, making it ideal for low-impact workouts.

Try standing on one leg or doing mild leg lifts in the water. The resistance of the water gives an added challenge to your balancing attempts while protecting your joints.

**2. *Slacklining:*** Slacklining is walking or balancing on a suspended stretch of flat webbing, comparable to tightrope walking but closer to the ground.

It involves regular balance adjustments and works your core, leg muscles, and stabilizers. Setting up a slackline in your garden or a local park may make balancing training more enjoyable and difficult.

**3. *Bosu Ball Exercises:*** The Bosu ball is a half-dome stability ball with a flat platform on the opposite side. Use the Bosu ball to do workouts such as squats, lunges, and standing balances.

The uneven surface challenges your body to use smaller stabilizing muscles, which improves joint stability and general balance.

**4. Animal Flow:** This bodyweight training approach uses primordial movements inspired by animals. It blends gymnastics, yoga, and breakdancing to create a fluid and dynamic exercise.

Many Animal Flow motions, such as beast crawls and crab reaches, demand balance and coordination, making them an efficient technique to enhance joint stability in a novel and fascinating way.

**5. Slackline Yoga**: Enjoy the advantages of slacklining and yoga in a peaceful outdoor setting, challenging your balance and flexibility. Practicing yoga postures on a slackline adds another level of difficulty, necessitating considerable attention and concentration to maintain balance.

Slackline yoga not only improves joint stability but also promotes mindfulness and body awareness.

**6. _Martial Arts:_** Tai Chi, Aikido, and Capoeira promote balance, agility, and coordination. These activities provide a comprehensive approach to joint stability by combining regulated motions, breathing methods, and mental focus.

Whether you practice slow, methodical movements in Tai Chi or fast, flowing motions in Capoeira, martial arts can help you improve your balance and general joint health.

Incorporating these novel and innovative balancing exercises into your training program may liven up your workouts while also improving joint stability.

With devotion and consistency, you'll benefit from better balance, a lower chance of injury, and a higher overall sense of well-being.

# *Isometric Exercises - Strengthening Muscles without Joint Stress*

Isometric exercises are a strong yet low-impact way to increase strength and muscle tone without putting undue strain on joints. Isometric workouts are especially good for men who want to increase their fitness without exacerbating joint problems.

They target muscles without the requirement for dynamic movement. Here's a detailed summary of isometric workouts and their advantages for men:

### What are isometric exercises?

Isometric workouts include tightening muscles while maintaining their length or joint angle. Unlike dynamic workouts, which require joint movement, isometric exercises use static postures, making them appropriate for men who have joint problems. These workouts may be done almost anyplace with minimum equipment, making them accessible and handy for people of all fitness levels.

**Advantages of Isometric Exercises for Men:**

**Strength Development:** Isometric workouts effectively activate muscle fibers, resulting in strength improvements. Men can improve muscle strength while maintaining static positions against resistance, avoiding joint stress.

**Joint Health:** Unlike high-impact workouts, isometric motions reduce joint strain. Men with joint problems or who are healing from traumas can safely develop their muscles without aggravating their pre-existing disorders.

Isometric exercises are ideal for efficient workouts since they need less time to complete. Men with hectic schedules can integrate isometric exercises into their workouts for short and efficient strength training sessions.

***Versatility:*** Isometric exercises may target many muscle groups, resulting in a complete full-body workout. Individual fitness objectives may be met with a variety of workouts ranging from core stability to upper and lower body strength development.

***Increased muscular Endurance:*** Static postures test muscular endurance, which improves stamina and resilience. Men can enhance their capacity to engage in sustained physical activity, whether for sports, work, or daily activities.

***Examples of isometric exercises:***

***Plank:*** The plank is a traditional core-strengthening exercise in which you hold a push-up posture with your body in a straight line from head to heels. This exercise works the abdominals, arms, shoulders, and back muscles.

The wall sit, performed with the back against a wall and the legs bent at a 90-degree angle works the quadriceps, hamstrings, and gluteus muscles. This position strengthens the lower body without putting stress on the knees or hips.

***Static Push-Up Hold:*** Holding the middle of a push-up with arms outstretched works the chest, shoulders, and triceps. This workout increases upper-body strength without the need for repetitive movement.

***Isometric Squat:*** Holding a squat position with thighs parallel to the ground works the quadriceps, hamstrings, and glutes. This exercise improves lower-body strength and stability without putting undue strain on the knees.

Isometric exercises are an effective and low-impact way to build muscles without causing joint stress, making them an excellent alternative for men looking to increase their fitness while limiting the chance of injury.

Men who incorporate isometric exercises into their regimens can acquire substantial strength, improve joint health, and get the advantages of a diverse and time-efficient workout plan.

# *Chapter 7: Mind-Body Connection in Low Impact Exercise*

Low-impact workouts are a mild but efficient technique for men to enhance their physical fitness while putting less strain on their joints and muscles.

Beyond the physical advantages, low-impact workouts promote a strong mind-body connection. Here's an in-depth look at how low-impact activities promote this link and why they're especially good for guys.

### *Understanding Low-Impact Exercises:*

Low-impact workouts are activities that place less strain on the joints, making them perfect for men of all ages and fitness levels, particularly those recuperating from injury or experiencing joint pain. These exercises usually include motions that keep at least one foot in contact with the ground at all times, which lowers the risk of impact-related injuries.

### Mind-Body Connection:

Low-impact workouts encourage males to be more aware of their motions. Walking, swimming, cycling, and yoga are examples of low-impact activities that emphasize controlled, deliberate motions, as opposed to high-impact workouts that need fast, powerful movements.

This emphasis on deliberate movement builds a stronger link between the mind and body, resulting in increased bodily awareness and control.

***Benefits for men:***

*__Tension Reduction:__* Low-impact workouts allow men to relax and relieve tension. Activities such as tai chi or mild stretching can help relieve stress in both the body and the mind, encouraging relaxation and mental clarity.

*__Improved Joint Health:__* Men are more susceptible to joint problems, especially as they age. Low-impact workouts allow you to develop the muscles that surround your joints without putting them under too much stress. This can help lower the risk of osteoarthritis and enhance overall joint function.

*__Improved Mental Health:__* Regular low-impact exercise has been related to higher mood and mental well-being. Walking and swimming, for example, have a rhythmic, repetitive character that helps relax the mind and reduce feelings of anxiety and sadness.

**Increased Flexibility and Mobility:** Many low-impact workouts aim to improve flexibility and mobility, which are critical components of overall fitness. Gentle stretching exercises and activities such as yoga can help men maintain or enhance their range of motion, making daily chores simpler and lowering their risk of injury.

**Long-Term Sustainability:** Unlike high-impact activities, which can harm the body over time, low-impact workouts are typically sustainable in the long run. Men can continue to benefit from these activities far into their retirement years, boosting longevity and preserving general health and vigor.

Low-impact workouts build a mind-body connection that is beneficial for men who want to enhance their physical fitness while focusing on joint health and mental well-being. Men may enjoy a comprehensive approach to exercise by including these moderate yet effective workouts into their daily regimen.

# Mindfulness Meditation for Stress Reduction

Stress has become a prevalent disease for many people, particularly males who are often pressured by society to present a strong exterior. However, stress management is critical for general well-being, and mindfulness meditation is gaining popularity as an effective technique.

Unlike strenuous physical activities, mindfulness meditation provides a low-impact yet potent method of stress reduction, making it a great practice for men who want to reduce stress while maintaining their physical health.

Mindfulness meditation entails establishing a state of concentrated awareness in the present moment, free of judgment or attachment to fleeting ideas or feelings. This technique enables people to notice their thoughts and feelings objectively, resulting in a sense of inner calm and clarity.

Mindfulness meditation, with continuous practice, can help remodel the brain by lowering reactivity in the amygdala—the brain's fear center—and increasing activity in areas linked with emotional control and self-awareness.

Men who are used to high-intensity workouts may find it difficult to incorporate mindfulness meditation into their daily practice at first. However, its simplicity and versatility make it suitable for people of all fitness levels.

Unlike intense physical exercises that might worsen current stress or exhaustion, mindfulness meditation provides a soothing alternative that revitalizes both the body and the mind.

One of the primary advantages of mindfulness meditation is its capacity to elicit a relaxation response—a state of profound rest that counteracts the stress reaction.

Men can benefit from this physiological transition by experiencing less muscular tension, lower blood pressure, and enhanced immunological function, which strengthens their resilience to stress-related health conditions.

Mindfulness meditation improves self-awareness, allowing men to identify early indicators of stress and respond before it worsens. Individuals can gain control over their reactions by being more aware of their thoughts and emotions, reducing the influence of stress on their general well-being.

Incorporating mindfulness meditation into a daily practice takes little time investment, making it accessible to even the busiest persons. Consistent practice of mindfulness meditation, whether for a few minutes in the morning or as a quick break during the day, can offer tremendous advantages over time.

Men can begin their mindfulness meditation practice with easy techniques like focused breathing or body scan activities. They can gradually include other mindfulness practices, such as mindful walking or loving-kindness meditation, to develop their practice and broaden their arsenal of stress-reduction skills.

Mindfulness meditation provides men with a comprehensive approach to stress reduction that compliments their current exercise program. By building present-moment awareness and emotional resilience, mindfulness meditation enables men to face life's problems with greater comfort and tranquility. Mindfulness meditation, as an accessible and low-impact practice, is an excellent tool for men looking to improve their general well-being and energy.

# Breathing Techniques for Relaxation and Focus

Stress and distractions may quickly overwhelm us, resulting in diminished productivity and general well-being. Fortunately, including breathing methods into your regular practice may bring significant advantages for both relaxation and attention.

These approaches, based on ancient traditions such as yoga and meditation, are simple yet effective tools for establishing a quiet and focused frame of mind. Incorporating breathing methods into low-impact activities might be especially useful for men looking for mental clarity and relaxation.

**1. Diaphragmatic Breathing:** Diaphragmatic breathing, also known as deep belly breathing, is the practice of

taking deep, slow breaths by activating the diaphragm.
 To perform this method, sit or lie down in a comfortable position.

With one hand on your abdomen, place the other hand on your chest.

As you fill your lungs with air, gently let your stomach expand.

As you fill your lungs with air and letting your stomach to expand,Inhale deeply through your nose

Exhale gently through your lips, feeling your abdominal muscles tense.

Concentrate on the rhythm of your breathing, letting any tension to release with each exhale.

**2. *Box Breathing:*** Box breathing is a simple yet powerful method for increasing relaxation and attention. Start by breathing deeply through your nose for a count of four. Hold your breath for four counts before gently exhaling through your lips for four counts.

Finally, wait for a count of four before starting the following cycle. Visualize drawing the shape of a square with each breath, focusing on equal durations for each phase. Repeat this practice for several minutes, progressively increasing the time as you get more familiar with the technique.

**3. *Alternate Nostril Breathing:*** This ancient yogic technique helps to balance the body's energies and relax the mind. Sit in a comfortable position, spine straight. Close your right nostril with your thumb and take a deep breath in through your left. At the top of your inhalation, shut your left nostril with your right ring finger, then release your thumb and exhale via your right nostril. Inhale via the right nostril, shut it with your thumb, and exhale through the left nostril. Repeat this pattern for many rounds, concentrating on the calm, even flow of your breath.

Incorporating these breathing methods into your regular practice can help you achieve a better feeling of serenity, attention, and general health. Whether you're struggling with work-related stress, navigating difficult situations, or simply looking for a moment of relaxation, these techniques can help you achieve inner calm and mental clarity.

Remember to approach each method with patience and attention, allowing yourself to fully experience the present moment and the healing power of your breath.

## Incorporating Mindful Movement into Your Exercise Routine

Exploring Mindful Movement Hiking is a terrific way to incorporate mindfulness into your outdoor workout regimen. Instead of hurrying along the trails, take your time and appreciate the sights, sounds, and fragrances of nature.

Pay attention to your breathing and the sense of the ground under you. Hiking thoughtfully gives not just physical exercise, but also mental renewal and a stronger connection to nature.

***Trail Running:*** For guys searching for a more dynamic kind of exercise, trail running is a fantastic way to develop mindful movement. Instead of focusing simply on pace and distance, consider your body's motions, breath rhythm, and changing terrain. Trail running provides a full-body exercise while immersing yourself in the beauty of the natural environment.

***Outdoor Yoga or Tai Chi:*** Extend your yoga or tai chi practice outside to reap the advantages of nature. Find a calm area in a park or near a lake to perform moderate stretches, postures, and movements. Allow the sounds of birds singing and the sensation of the air on your skin to deepen your meditation and strengthen your connection with nature.

***Kayaking or Canoeing:*** Practice mindful movement while exploring bodies of water by kayaking or canoeing. Concentrate on the rhythmic action of paddling, the sensation of water beneath your feet, and the sights and sounds of the surrounding environment. These exercises not only give a low-impact workout but also allow for rest and reflection.

Outdoor Meditation: To incorporate mindfulness meditation into your outdoor workout program, choose a peaceful location in nature to sit and contemplate.

Close your eyes, concentrate on your breathing, and allow yourself to be completely present in the moment. Embrace the sounds of nature and the warmth of the sun on your skin as you create inner serenity and calm.

Men may improve their fitness regimen and enjoy the many advantages of nature by adding mindful movement to outdoor activities.

Whether hiking, trail jogging, practicing yoga or tai chi outside, or participating in water sports, the objective is to stay present in the moment, which allows for a deeper connection with both the body and the environment.

# CONCLUSION

Low-impact activities have several benefits for men, catering to all fitness levels and health concerns. Walking, swimming, cycling, and yoga are examples of moderate yet effective workouts that may promote general health and well-being without placing too much strain on the body.

To begin, men of all ages and fitness levels can participate in low-impact workouts. They provide a starting point for newcomers as well as a long-term solution for individuals recuperating from injuries or managing chronic diseases.

Walking or swimming can help men gradually improve strength, endurance, and flexibility while lowering the risk of injury associated with high-impact sports.

Furthermore, low-impact activities are beneficial to cardiovascular health. Cycling and swimming increase the heart rate, which improves circulation and lowers blood pressure.

These activities help improve lung function, increasing oxygen uptake and general respiratory health. Men who incorporate regular low-impact exercise into their routines can lower their risk of heart disease, stroke, and other cardiovascular disorders.

Low-impact workouts also help to preserve joint health and mobility. Low-impact workouts, such as yoga and Pilates, enhance flexibility, balance, and range of motion without putting undue load on the joints.
This is especially good for elderly men or those with joint diseases such as arthritis,

as it relieves pain and stiffness while maintaining joint function over time.

Low-impact workouts promote general mental health. Yoga and tai chi are two hobbies that promote relaxation and awareness, which can help to alleviate stress, anxiety, and depression.

Regular exercise produces endorphins, neurotransmitters that improve mood and lessen pain and suffering. Men who incorporate low-impact activities into their daily regimen might benefit from increased mental clarity, mood, and stress management.

Low-impact activities are a safe, effective, and easily accessible option for men to enhance their physical and mental health. Men may get the many advantages of exercise while reducing their risk of injury and strain by including activities such as walking, swimming, cycling, and yoga into their daily routine. Low-impact activities are a versatile and long-term option for men of all ages and fitness levels, whether they are looking to improve cardiovascular health, preserve joint function, or improve general wellness.

# *THANK YOU PAGE*

Thank you for selecting this book. Your support is really appreciated. Similarly, I am grateful for the purchase of this book.

Your input is valuable; please share your ideas in a review. It serves as a reference for future improvements. Enjoy reading and utilizing it!

# Workout planner to help track Progress

## Workout Planner

Week : _______________

Month: _______________

Sunday          Monday          Tuesday

Goals           Goals           **Goals**

Wednesday          Thursday          Friday

Goals           **Goals**           Goals

Saturday

Goals                    Mood

Motivation _______________________________
_________________________________________
_________________________________________
_________________________________________
_________________________________________
_________________________________________

## Workout Planner

Week : _______________

Month: _______________

Sunday

Monday

Tuesday

Goals

Goals

**Goals**

Wednesday

Thursday

Friday

Goals

**Goals**

Goals

Saturday

Goals

Goals

Mood

Motivation _______________

## WEEKLY

*Workout Planner*

Week : _______________

Month: _______________

Sunday            Monday            Tuesday

| Goals | Goals | **Goals** |

Wednesday         Thursday          Friday

| Goals | **Goals** | Goals |

Saturday

| Goals | Mood |

Motivation _______________________
_________________________________
_________________________________
_________________________________
_________________________________

# Workout Planner

Week : _______________

Month: _______________

Sunday | Monday | Tuesday

| Goals | Goals | **Goals** |

Wednesday | Thursday | Friday

| Goals | **Goals** | Goals |

Saturday

| Goals | Mood |

Motivation _______________

_______________

_______________

_______________

_______________

**WEEKLY** *Workout Planner*

Week : ______________

Month: ______________

Sunday

Monday

Tuesday

Goals

Goals

**Goals**

Wednesday

Thursday

Friday

Goals

**Goals**

Goals

Saturday

Goals

*Mood*

Motivation __________________

Workout Planner

Week : ______________

Month: ______________

Sunday

Monday

Tuesday

Goals

Goals

Goals

Wednesday

Thursday

Friday

Goals

Goals

Goals

Saturday

Goals

Mood

Motivation ___________________________
_______________________________________
_______________________________________
_______________________________________
_______________________________________

# WEEKLY

## Workout Planner

Week : _______________

Month: _______________

Sunday

Monday

Tuesday

Goals

Goals

**Goals**

Wednesday

Thursday

Friday

Goals

**Goals**

Goals

Saturday

Goals

Mood

Motivation _______________

# Workout Planner

Week : _______________

Month: _______________

Sunday

Monday

Tuesday

Goals

Goals

**Goals**

Wednesday

Thursday

Friday

Goals

**Goals**

Goals

Saturday

Goals

Mood

Motivation _______________

Workout Planner

Week :_____________

Month: _____________

Sunday

Monday

Tuesday

Goals

Goals

Goals

Wednesday

Thursday

Friday

Goals

Goals

Goals

Saturday

Goals

Mood

Motivation ___________________________
_____________________________________
_____________________________________
_____________________________________
_____________________________________

# Workout Planner

Week : _______________

Month: _______________

Sunday

Monday

Tuesday

Goals

Goals

**Goals**

Wednesday

Thursday

Friday

Goals

**Goals**

Goals

Saturday

Goals

Mood

Motivation _______________

## Workout Planner

**Week :** _______________

**Month:** _______________

Sunday          Monday          Tuesday

| Goals | Goals | Goals |

Wednesday       Thursday        Friday

| Goals | Goals | Goals |

Saturday

| Goals | Mood |

Motivation _______________

_______________________________________

_______________________________________

_______________________________________

_______________________________________

# Workout Planner

Week : _______________

Month: _______________

**WEEKLY**

Sunday          Monday          Tuesday

| Goals | Goals | **Goals** |

Wednesday       Thursday        Friday

| Goals | **Goals** | Goals |

Saturday

| Goals | Mood |

Motivation ___________________
___________________________
___________________________
___________________________
___________________________
___________________________

Workout Planner

**WEEKLY**

Week : _______________

Month: _______________

Sunday

Monday

Tuesday

Goals

Goals

**Goals**

Wednesday

Thursday

Friday

Goals

**Goals**

Goals

Saturday

Goals

Mood

Motivation _______________
_______________________________
_______________________________
_______________________________
_______________________________
_______________________________

## Workout Planner

Week : _______________

Month: _______________

Sunday

Monday

Tuesday

Goals

Goals

**Goals**

Wednesday

Thursday

Friday

Goals

**Goals**

Goals

Saturday

Goals

Mood

Motivation _______________________________

## Workout Planner

**WEEKLY**

Week : _______________

Month: _______________

Sunday

Monday

Tuesday

Goals

Goals

**Goals**

Wednesday

Thursday

Friday

Goals

**Goals**

Goals

Saturday

Goals

Mood

Motivation _______________

## Workout Planner

**Week :** ___________

**Month:** ___________

Sunday

Monday

Tuesday

Goals

Goals

**Goals**

Wednesday

Thursday

Friday

Goals

Goals

Goals

Saturday

Goals

Mood

Motivation ________________________________

________________________________________

________________________________________

________________________________________

________________________________________

________________________________________

WEEKLY

*Workout Planner*

Week : ______________

Month: ______________

Sunday

Monday

Tuesday

Goals

Goals

Goals

Wednesday

Thursday

Friday

Goals

Goals

Goals

Saturday

Goals

Mood

Motivation ________________________________
________________________________
________________________________
________________________________
________________________________
________________________________

# Workout Planner

Week :_________________

Month: _______________

Sunday

Monday

Tuesday

Goals

Goals

**Goals**

Wednesday

Thursday

Friday

Goals

Goals

Goals

Saturday

Goals

Mood

Motivation _______________________

WEEKLY

*Workout Planner*

Week : ______________

Month: ______________

Sunday

Monday

Tuesday

Goals

Goals

**Goals**

Wednesday

Thursday

Friday

Goals

**Goals**

Goals

Saturday

Goals

Mood

Motivation _______________________________

## Workout Planner

Week : _______________

Month: _______________

Sunday

Monday

Tuesday

| Goals | Goals | **Goals** |

Wednesday

Thursday

Friday

| Goals | **Goals** | Goals |

Saturday

| Goals | Mood |

Motivation _______________

_______________________________

_______________________________

_______________________________

_______________________________

_______________________________

# WEEKLY

## Workout Planner

Week : ___________________

Month: ________________

Sunday

Monday

Tuesday

Goals

Goals

**Goals**

Wednesday

Thursday

Friday

Goals

Goals

Goals

Saturday

Goals

Mood

Motivation ___________________

Workout Planner

Week : _________________

Month: _________________

Sunday          Monday          Tuesday

Goals          Goals          **Goals**

Wednesday          Thursday          Friday

Goals          **Goals**          Goals

Saturday

Goals          Mood

Motivation __________________________
________________________________________
________________________________________
________________________________________
________________________________________

## Workout Planner

Week : ___________

Month: ___________

Sunday          Monday          Tuesday

| Goals | Goals | Goals |

Wednesday       Thursday        Friday

| Goals | Goals | Goals |

Saturday

| Goals | Mood |

Motivation ___________________________

_____________________________________

_____________________________________

_____________________________________

_____________________________________

# Workout Planner

Week : _______________

Month: _______________

Sunday

Monday

Tuesday

Goals

Goals

Goals

Wednesday

Thursday

Friday

Goals

Goals

Goals

Saturday

Goals

Mood

Motivation _______________

## Workout Planner

Week : ___________________

Month: ___________________

Sunday

Monday

Tuesday

Goals

Goals

**Goals**

Wednesday

Thursday

Friday

Goals

Goals

Goals

Saturday

Goals

Mood

Motivation ________________________________

____________________________________________

____________________________________________

____________________________________________

____________________________________________

**WEEKLY**

*Workout Planner*

Week : _______________

Month: _______________

Sunday          Monday          Tuesday

| Goals | Goals | **Goals** |

Wednesday       Thursday        Friday

| Goals | **Goals** | Goals |

Saturday

| Goals | Mood |

Motivation _______________________________
_________________________________________
_________________________________________
_________________________________________
_________________________________________

Sunday     Monday     Tuesday

Goals     Goals     **Goals**

Wednesday     Thursday     Friday

Goals     **Goals**     Goals

Saturday

Goals     Mood

Motivation _______________________________

WEEKLY

Workout Planner

Week : _______________

Month: _______________

Sunday

Monday

Tuesday

Goals

Goals

Goals

Wednesday

Thursday

Friday

Goals

Goals

Goals

Saturday

Goals

Mood

Motivation _______________________________

________________________________________

________________________________________

________________________________________

________________________________________

## WEEKLY

## Workout Planner

Week : _______________

Month: _______________

Sunday          Monday          Tuesday

| Goals | Goals | Goals |

Wednesday       Thursday        Friday

| Goals | Goals | Goals |

Saturday

| Goals | Mood |

Motivation _______________

_______________________________________

_______________________________________

_______________________________________

_______________________________________

Workout Planner

Week :______________

Month: ______________

Sunday

Monday

Tuesday

Goals

Goals

Goals

Wednesday

Thursday

Friday

Goals

Goals

Goals

Saturday

Goals

Mood

Motivation __________________

Workout Planner

Week : _______________

Month: _______________

Sunday

Monday

Tuesday

Goals

Goals

Goals

Wednesday

Thursday

Friday

Goals

Goals

Goals

Saturday

Goals

Mood

Motivation _______________

## Workout Planner

WEEKLY

Week : _______________

Month: _______________

Sunday

Monday

Tuesday

Goals

Goals

Goals

Wednesday

Thursday

Friday

Goals

Goals

Goals

Saturday

Goals

Mood

Motivation _______________________________

Workout Planner

Week : _______________

Month: _______________

WEEKLY

Sunday

Monday

Tuesday

Goals

Goals

**Goals**

Wednesday

Thursday

Friday

Goals

**Goals**

Goals

Saturday

Goals

Mood

Motivation _____________________________
_________________________________________
_________________________________________
_________________________________________
_________________________________________
_________________________________________

# WEEKLY

## Workout Planner

Week : _______________

Month: _______________

Sunday

Monday

Tuesday

Goals

Goals

**Goals**

Wednesday

Thursday

Friday

Goals

**Goals**

Goals

Saturday

Goals

Mood

Motivation _______________

Sunday

Monday

Tuesday

Goals

Goals

Goals

Wednesday

Thursday

Friday

Goals

Goals

Goals

Saturday

Goals

Mood

Motivation ________________________

## Workout Planner

Week : ___________________

Month: ___________________

Sunday

Monday

Tuesday

Goals

Goals

**Goals**

Wednesday

Thursday

Friday

Goals

**Goals**

Goals

Saturday

Goals

Mood

Motivation _______________________

## Workout Planner

Week :______________

Month: ______________

Sunday

Monday

Tuesday

Goals

Goals

**Goals**

Wednesday

Thursday

Friday

Goals

Goals

Goals

Saturday

Goals

Mood

Motivation ______________

Workout Planner

Week :______________

Month: ______________

WEEKLY

Sunday

Monday

Tuesday

Goals

Goals

**Goals**

Wednesday

Thursday

Friday

Goals

**Goals**

Goals

Saturday

Goals

Mood

Motivation ________________________________

## Workout Planner

Week : ___________________

Month: ___________________

Sunday

Monday

Tuesday

Goals

Goals

**Goals**

Wednesday

Thursday

Friday

Goals

**Goals**

Goals

Saturday

Goals

Mood

Motivation ___________________

# Workout Planner

Weekly

Week: ___________

Month: ___________

| Sunday | Monday | Tuesday |
|--------|--------|---------|
| Goals | Goals | **Goals** |

| Wednesday | Thursday | Friday |
|-----------|----------|--------|
| Goals | **Goals** | Goals |

| Saturday | Mood |
|----------|------|
| Goals | |

Motivation ________________________________
______________________________________________
______________________________________________
______________________________________________
______________________________________________

## Workout Planner

Week :_______________

Month:_____________

Sunday

Monday

Tuesday

Goals

Goals

Goals

Wednesday

Thursday

Friday

Goals

Goals

Goals

Saturday

Goals

Mood

Motivation _______________

## Workout Planner

Weekly

Week : _____________

Month: _____________

Sunday

Monday

Tuesday

Goals

Goals

Goals

Wednesday

Thursday

Friday

Goals

Goals

Goals

Saturday

Goals

Mood

Motivation _________________________
_______________________________________
_______________________________________
_______________________________________
_______________________________________
_______________________________________

# WEEKLY

## Workout Planner

Week : ___________

Month: ___________

Sunday

Monday

Tuesday

| Goals | Goals | **Goals** |

Wednesday

Thursday

Friday

| Goals | Goals | Goals |

Saturday

| Goals | Mood |

Motivation ______________________________
______________________________
______________________________
______________________________
______________________________
______________________________

# Workout Planner

**WEEKLY**

Week : _______________

Month: _______________

Sunday

Monday

Tuesday

| Goals | Goals | **Goals** |

Wednesday

Thursday

Friday

| Goals | **Goals** | Goals |

Saturday

| Goals | | Mood |

Motivation _______________________________

_______________________________________

_______________________________________

_______________________________________

_______________________________________

WEEKLY

Workout Planner

Week : _______________

Month: _______________

Sunday          Monday          Tuesday

Goals           Goals           **Goals**

Wednesday       Thursday        Friday

Goals           **Goals**       Goals

Saturday

Goals           Mood

Motivation _______________________________
___________________________________________
___________________________________________
___________________________________________
___________________________________________
___________________________________________

# Workout Planner

Weekly

Week : ___________

Month: ___________

Sunday          Monday          Tuesday

| Goals | Goals | Goals |

Wednesday       Thursday        Friday

| Goals | Goals | Goals |

Saturday

| Goals | Mood |

Motivation ________________________________
_____________________________________________
_____________________________________________
_____________________________________________
_____________________________________________
_____________________________________________

## Workout Planner

Sunday        Monday        Tuesday

| Goals | Goals | **Goals** |

Wednesday     Thursday      Friday

| Goals | **Goals** | Goals |

Saturday

| Goals | Mood |

Motivation ________________________
___________________________________
___________________________________
___________________________________
___________________________________

# Workout Planner

Week : _______________

Month: _______________

Sunday     Monday     Tuesday

| Goals | Goals | Goals |

Wednesday     Thursday     Friday

| Goals | Goals | Goals |

Saturday

| Goals | Mood |

Motivation _______________

## Workout Planner

Week : ___________

Month: ___________

Sunday

Monday

Tuesday

Goals

Goals

**Goals**

Wednesday

Thursday

Friday

Goals

**Goals**

Goals

Saturday

Goals

Mood

Motivation ________________________________

## Workout Planner

Week : _______________

Month: _______________

Sunday

Monday

Tuesday

Goals

Goals

Goals

Wednesday

Thursday

Friday

Goals

Goals

Goals

Saturday

Goals

Mood

Motivation _______________

WEEKLY

Workout Planner

Week : ______________

Month: ______________

Sunday    Monday    Tuesday

Goals    Goals    **Goals**

Wednesday    Thursday    Friday

Goals    **Goals**    Goals

Saturday

Goals    Mood

Motivation ______________________________
___________________________________________
___________________________________________
___________________________________________
___________________________________________
___________________________________________

# Workout Planner

WEEKLY

Week : _______________

Month: _______________

Sunday

Monday

Tuesday

| Goals | Goals | Goals |

Wednesday

Thursday

Friday

| Goals | Goals | Goals |

Saturday

| Goals |

Mood

Motivation _______________

# Workout Planner

Week : _______________

Month: _______________

Sunday

Monday

Tuesday

Goals

Goals

**Goals**

Wednesday

Thursday

Friday

Goals

**Goals**

Goals

Saturday

Goals

Mood

Motivation _______________

## Workout Planner

Week : _____________

Month: _____________

Sunday

Monday

Tuesday

| Goals | Goals | **Goals** |

Wednesday

Thursday

Friday

| Goals | **Goals** | Goals |

Saturday

| Goals | Mood |

Motivation ________________________

## WEEKLY

Workout Planner

Week :_______________

Month: _______________

Sunday

Monday

Tuesday

Goals

Goals

Goals

Wednesday

Thursday

Friday

Goals

Goals

Goals

Saturday

Goals

Mood

Motivation _______________

## Workout Planner

Week : _______________

Month: _______________

Sunday

Monday

Tuesday

Goals

Goals

**Goals**

Wednesday

Thursday

Friday

Goals

**Goals**

Goals

Saturday

Goals

Mood

Motivation _______________

# Workout Planner

Weekly

Week : _____________

Month: _____________

Sunday

Monday

Tuesday

Goals

Goals

Goals

Wednesday

Thursday

Friday

Goals

Goals

Goals

Saturday

Goals

Mood

Motivation _____________________________

# Workout Planner

Week : _______________

Month: _______________

Sunday

Monday

Tuesday

Goals

Goals

Goals

Wednesday

Thursday

Friday

Goals

Goals

Goals

Saturday

Goals

Mood

Motivation _______________
_______________________________
_______________________________
_______________________________
_______________________________

## Workout Planner

**Week :** _______________

**Month:** _______________

WEEKLY

Sunday

Monday

Tuesday

Goals

Goals

Goals

Wednesday

Thursday

Friday

Goals

Goals

Goals

Saturday

Goals

Mood

Motivation _______________

## Workout Planner

Week : _______________

Month: _______________

Sunday

Monday

Tuesday

Goals

Goals

**Goals**

Wednesday

Thursday

Friday

Goals

Goals

Goals

Saturday

Goals

Mood

Motivation _______________

## Workout Planner

Week : __________________

Month: __________________

Sunday          Monday          Tuesday

Goals          Goals          **Goals**

Wednesday          Thursday          Friday

Goals          **Goals**          Goals

Saturday

Goals          Mood

Motivation ______________________________

________________________________________

________________________________________

________________________________________

________________________________________

# Workout Planner

Week : _______________

Month: _______________

Sunday

Monday

Tuesday

Goals

Goals

**Goals**

Wednesday

Thursday

Friday

Goals

**Goals**

Goals

Saturday

Goals

Mood

Motivation _______________

# Workout Planner

Week : _______________

Month: _______________

Sunday

Monday

Tuesday

Goals

Goals

**Goals**

Wednesday

Thursday

Friday

Goals

**Goals**

Goals

Saturday

Goals

Mood

Motivation ________________________________
________________________________
________________________________
________________________________
________________________________

## Workout Planner

**Week :** _______________

**Month:** _______________

| Sunday | Monday | Tuesday |
|---|---|---|
| Goals | Goals | Goals |

| Wednesday | Thursday | Friday |
|---|---|---|
| Goals | Goals | Goals |

Saturday

Goals

Mood

Motivation _______________________________

________________________________________

________________________________________

________________________________________

________________________________________

Workout Planner

Week :_______________

Month: _______________

WEEKLY

Sunday

Monday

Tuesday

Goals

Goals

Goals

Wednesday

Thursday

Friday

Goals

Goals

Goals

Saturday

Goals

Mood

Motivation ___________________________

# Workout Planner

**WEEKLY**

Week : ___________

Month: ___________

Sunday

Monday

Tuesday

Goals

Goals

**Goals**

Wednesday

Thursday

Friday

Goals

**Goals**

Goals

Saturday

Goals

Mood

Motivation ___________